GOT PROTOCOLS?

THE INSIDER'S GUIDE

to creating lucrative and efficient protocols that will change your medical practice

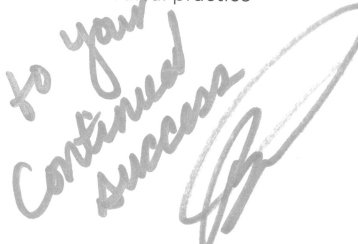

to your Continued success

HOLLY BURKMAN

ISBN: 9781698980850

Printed in USA

Cover Design by Justin Hook

Interior Design by Najdan Mancic

CONTENTS

FOREWORD

———————

This book is a goldmine of information. Holly uses a no-nonsense approach with proven results. There is no fluff. All the information included can be implemented in your office, if you are serious about having a successful practice and streamlining your clinic.

Writing an invitation for a book about medical business protocols is both intimidating and exciting at the same time. If you asked me 10 years ago to write a foreword I would have been overwhelmed and frustrated but not at all excited.

Medicine is an ever changing and evolving field. Every medical textbook has this disclaimer. None of our medical school training prepares us for the reality of life and the business of medicine. Like it or not, the real world has moved from the art of medicine to the business of medicine. We as physicians need to change with the times. We are first business owners and second physicians.

During the initial years of my practice, I used to hate the words customers, clients or members instead of patients. I avoided looking at them as customers and refused to think of my practice as a business, however, I have been wrong from the beginning. Over time I realized that at the end of the day, a medical practice is a business and patients are our clients. We have a duty to provide comprehensive affordable care to our patients. This only occurs when we implement sound protocols in our office.

In this book you will see the words "change", "family", "happiness" all which are the most vital part of your life. Do not allow medicine to consume your life and get burned out. In this book there is vital information on how to practice good medicine and not have it consume your life.

It is imperative for all of you to make an effort to really devour this book. Use an open mind and see how much it can change your practice for good. Give it a month, preferably 6 months and you will start seeing the difference. Holly is a genius, who I wish, I had met much earlier in my practice and not spent countless nights thinking about finances and multiple hours charting in the EMR.

Lastly, I would like to congratulate Holly for putting all her thoughts on paper as it is very hard sometimes to bring those hard topics to the front. It is hard for you to admit that you have a problem in your practice, but change is the only way to survive in this era of medicine without burning yourself out.

Karanvir Virk M.D.

Why Bother With Change?

One day.

Physicians want their medical practices to change, one day.

One day they will not spend weekends doing documentation.

One day the office staff will not complain.

One day they will not have to yell down the hall for help

One day there will be enough money in the bank.

One day all patients will be compliant.

One day rooms will be set up correctly.

One day there will not be a crisis at work.

One day their staff will be happy.

One day they will be happy.

Physicians want their staff, practice, and lives to change. They want to make more money, take more vacations and have more time. They want a better work life balance. They want to practice they way they imagined. Yet, after running a medical practice for 5, 10, or even 20 years, reality hits.

Nothing will change.

Physicians talk about change. They want change and they dream about it. They attend conferences. They buy programs. They join Facebook groups thinking there is a magic pill that will make all their problems go away.

Still, nothing changes.

They dream, whine and drink more wine hoping that a change is on the horizon. Guess what? It will never change. You will never change.

It's all because of one little word:

Protocols.

CHAPTER ONE

Creating a Shift

· ·

▶ Why great doctors run inefficient practices

▶ What to do when passion fades

▶ Overcoming common office issues

· ·

W hen my husband and I started our medical practice, I never dreamed of the problems we would face — audits, insurance denials, accounting nightmares, staff recruitment and retention, endless paperwork, EMR and government regulation to name a few. What started out as an adventure quickly nose-dived into a nightmare.

I held the office together, playing almost every role: biller, front desk clerk, office manager, and HR director. At the time, my ability to buy groceries and pay the mortgage was dependent on what happened in the office. I had skin in the game; my family had skin in the game. My choices were to rise above the issues and find solutions or go down with the practice.

I choose to fix them.

Fast forward to today: our medical practice is a well-oiled machine. We have implemented *systems and protocols* that have completely changed the way our office functions. I never thought about the enormous implications of these changes until I started visiting other medical practices and realized how much practitioners were struggling. They desperately needed help to get beyond crisis mode — a plight I knew all too well.

Making a Change

While I still play an intregal part in my husband's practice, I spend most of my time working with physicians and improving their practices. Throughout the years, my experiences have made me selective about where I put my time and energy. I only work with a doctor if they are at a turning point; they must be ready to fight to make their practice better.

I refuse to work with people who don't **really** want to change. I don't have time to coddle a physician; they either truly want to fix their environment or they don't. **It's that simple**.

The most successful practices I have worked with are run by physicians who don't dread the forms I make them complete. Instead, they are filled out thoroughly and emailed back to me quickly. They are eager to meet with me and excited about new possibilities. They are ready to make changes. They are either at a crisis point or just excited at the possibility of running a smoother practice.

These physicians are the ones that I know will succeed. They have a passion and a desire to change, they just need direction.

Passion Equals Progress

When I begin the consultation process I ask a client what their passion is. Usually, they give me a perplexed look and answer with something along the lines of "helping people," "medicine," or some other equally lame answer. I roll my eyes and tell them to try again. Sputtering, the physicians have no idea what to say.

Their passion has disappeared. The spark is gone. They are in medicine but very few of them know why they are physicians. Instead of a calling, it is now just a job. It is a job that they need to pay the bills, to pay their employees. A job that they need to just keep their head above water. Their passion is gone.

All physicians were passionate when they entered medical school. They had to be. The rigors of schooling, financial commitment, and the grueling schedule would not have been possible if they were not 100% committed to their goals. However, at some point in the journey, they began to view their careers as a mere obligation—something they were no longer emotionally invested in—not the career they worked so hard to achieve.

People are quick to say that physicians are burnt out; that they need to renew themselves. But this is not what causes a lack of passion.

Many times, as a consultant, I go into the medical offices and I see doctors rushing from room to room trying to see as many patients as possible. In this process, they are thinking:

☑ I should have dispensed that brace.

☑ I have to remember to check her lab work.

☑ I should run that test.

☑ I need to remember to call that last patient.

☑ I should have used that ultrasound machine.

☑ I need to use that new thing I bought at the last conference.

☑ Did I meet the MIPS requirements?

☑ Where is my nurse?

☑ Where are my supplies?

☑ Crap, I'm running an hour behind and Mrs. Jones is waiting for me.

They frantically rush to the next room yelling at their medical assistants to bring them this or to do that. At the end of the day they sit down to three hours' worth of charting and a falling bank balance and think: "This is not why I went to medical school. This is not why I own a private practice. This is not what my life was supposed to be like," they tell themselves. "I am failing as a doctor and a business owner. What am I even doing here?"

> **If a physician cannot tell me *why* they are passionate about being a physician, their practice is in grave danger. A medical practice without passion cannot succeed!**

The long hours, high levels of emotional and monetary investment, and staff management can be exhaustive and discouraging.

Without passion, no one will survive this journey.

Without passion, physicians will *not* change.

Without change, practices will continue to be the same.

Without change, their protocols and procedures will never improve.

Without passion, a physician can not motivate, encourage or lead their staff.

In short, a practice without passion is doomed to fail.

Some physicians are stalled by fear of the unknown, but they still know that change MUST happen to stay in business. All they need is someone to push them to accomplish something they could only dream about.

In short, most physicians want to change but are unsure how to go about it.

Finding Answers

One of the biggest changes that I have implemented into medical practices is protocols. Every business in the world operates through protocols.

Think about it:

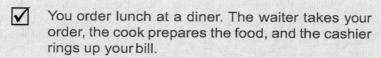

☑ You order lunch at a diner. The waiter takes your order, the cook prepares the food, and the cashier rings up your bill.

☑ You are greeted as you walk into a store. An associate helps you find the perfect shirt, and a clerk checks you out.

☑ You buy your movie ticket, go to the concession stand, and then you run to find your seat in the theater.

Whether private or in a public setting, protocols provide a sense of security and familiarity. They make systems run smoothly and control customer/client expectations. While you may only see a few things happening at the store or a movie theater, there are hundreds of protocols at work behind the scenes that you will never see or think about. If even one of those 'hidden' protocols is not completed, your experience won't be the same. Who inventories clothes? Who buys the merchandise? Who cleans the stores? Who buys the popcorn? Who cleans the machines? Who turns on the video projector? What would happen if there was no popcorn available, if your theater seat was dirty, or if the movie never started, your customer experience would be ruined.

Your practice is no different.

Protocols are the lifeblood of any medical practice.

Protocols allow:

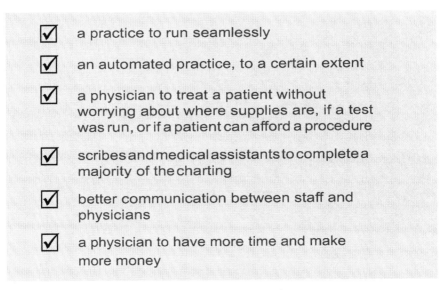

- ☑ a practice to run seamlessly
- ☑ an automated practice, to a certain extent
- ☑ a physician to treat a patient without worrying about where supplies are, if a test was run, or if a patient can afford a procedure
- ☑ scribes and medical assistants to complete a majority of the charting
- ☑ better communication between staff and physicians
- ☑ a physician to have more time and make more money

In a nutshell, **protocols transform practices.**

You say to yourself, wait, if I establish protocols won't I just be a trained robot mindlessly, following protocols? Where is the fun in that? Where is the adrenalin rush? Where is the satisfaction of diagnosing and treating my patients? Where is the fulfillment that comes from solving their medical problems and making them feel better? My practice may be driving me nuts, but I have no intention of becoming a trained robot. If I wanted to be told what to do and how to do it I would work for someone else.

Let me ask you this? How many patients that come in with a high fever and sore throat have a diagnosis of strep? It's predictable 95% of the time. So your protocol will work 95% of the time. What about the other 5% that don't fit in the mold? This is where your amazing abilities come in. This is where your treatment options change. This is where the magic is. If you are not rushed, if you are not yelling for this or that and/or upset because you forgot that test, you are able to free your mind, talk with your patients and catch those patients who present with that 5 % abnormality. If you are rushed and behind, it is easier to miss things that may change your diagnosis and therefore your treatment plan.

Protocols free up your time and your mind to allow you to be the physician you trained to be. Protocols do not make you a robot, they make you a more conscious physician.

Protocols vs. Protocols

My career is centered on implementing protocols in medical practices. Countless years have taught me that the way I produce protocols and the way physicians produce protocols are entirely different.

For physicians, they are tests and procedures

In medical school, students learn all about the steps to give an injection, do a throat swab, take blood pressure, perform CPR, and save a life. They understand these as "medical protocols." This is what a typical medical protocol looks like to a physician.

HEEL PAIN PROTOCOL

1. Calcaneal X-Rays of heel 2 view
2. Diagnose
3. Inject cortisone is neccesary

When I refer to protocols, I mean the *entire* process. This means there are clear guidelines attached to every step from the moment the phone is answered to the time the patient receives a bill for service. Every step of the process is integral to how a physician treats their patients and how a practice runs.

Every person's responsibility is clearly defined.

HEEL PAIN PROTOCOL #1
Phone Interaction when scheduling the visit:

Thank you for calling....
How can I help you?
Have you see Dr. ..... before?
Let me get some additional information to help me schedule you correctly.

- [x] NLDOCAT
  - Nature
  - Location
  - Duration
  - Onset
  - Course
  - Aggregating Factor
  - Previous Treatment
- [x] Insurance Information
- [x] Confirm Appointment Time
- [x] Check insurance coverage before the visit

Medical Assistant [20 minutes]:

- [x] Bring patient back
- [x] Take vitals
- [x] Update NLDOCAT
- [x] Perform procedures needed prior to doctor examination
  - ex: x-rays, blood work, etc.
- [x] Bring in heel pain kit
  - OCT
    - Plantar Sleeve
    - Samples of orthotics
  - Braces
  - Consent forms
  - Prepare information for the doctor
  - Upload x-rays
  - Draw up cortisone injection, set out gloves, alcohol, ultrasound machine
  - Start chart note, enter template

HEEL PAIN PROTOCOL #2
Doctor [10 Minutes]

- ☑ Examination
- ☑ Cortisone injection
- ☑ Talk with patient
- ☑ Possible orthotics and night splint

Medical Assistant [10 min]

- ☑ Review cost of orthotics and night splint.
- ☑ Give follow up instructions
- ☑ Sign proof of delivery forms/consent forms
- ☑ Walk the patient to the front desk
- ☑ Discuss all completed procedures and related cost with the front desk
- ☑ Drop off superbill and paperwork that needs to be scanned and uploaded

Front Desk Associate

- ☑ Process all monetary transactions: Collect against deductible and co-insurance
- ☑ Schedule follow up
- ☑ RTC: 2 weeks

Medical assistant

- ☑ Clean room
- ☑ Finish office note

Doctor

- ☑ Sign office note
- ☑ Send over billing

Compare the differences.

> The second set of protocols is much more comprehensive. It covers everything from job responsibility to appointment length to billing codes.

Without these types of protocols, physicians are too distracted by insufficient revenue, hindrances in communication, and managing staff. They can no longer focus on what they are trained to do: treat patients. They run from room to room, never being able to connect with the people they're serving. Instead, they are always worried about documentation, where the supplies are, and what they forgot to do.

These types of protocols allow everyone on the team to know exactly what to do and when. This creates an organized atmosphere.

Implementing protocols changes medical practices.

When physicians are unable to completely focus on their patients, both the patients and practice suffer. Physicians went to medical school to treat patients not to deal with the endless hours of documentation, HR nightmares, billing, and insurance regulations. You went to school to make a difference. You went to school to treat patients and build a fulfilling and meaningful career. But due to the endless regulations, frustration, communication breakdown, and office inefficiencies. Your passion starts to fade. You begin to wonder, why am I here? Why am I in private practice? Why am I a physician? There has to be a better way. *There is!* Building and implementing correctly structured protocols save practices and start to ignite the passion within the physician again.

Protocols can solve a whole myriad of problems, but they require time and energy to build. Most importantly they require change.

Change is difficult. One must be at a crossroads and ready to make the leap. Protocols are not a willy nilly thing. You either follow them or you don't. Don't waste time developing protocols if you are going to refuse to follow them and compel your staff to do the same. This is a waste of your time and adds to the frustration of yourself and your staff members. You can't change your protocols daily, you can't decide that today you will follow them and tomorrow you won't.

I help people solve problems. I find answers and solutions, and I am extremely good at it. However, I cannot make someone change. Change must come from within. It must be fueled by personal desire, passion, and motivation.

This book will explain why your past protocols have failed, and why new protocols are essential. The following chapters will provide you with a road map to building your own protocols that will change your practice. This will allow you to be the physician you went to school to be.

However, this book <u>will</u> require change. That part is up to you.

Are you willing to act on what this book guides you to do?

Will you put in the effort that this book will demand of you?

Are you willing to step outside of your comfort zone?

Are you willing to solve the problems that plague you?

Are you ready to be passionate about your business and life again?

Are you willing to make your practice successful?

Will this be day one, or are you still stuck on "one day"?

You Decide.

REFLECTION QUESTIONS

What is your passion?

What would get you up for (happily) at 4 a.m.?

What makes you smile?

What patients make you smile?

Why did you go to medical school?

CHAPTER TWO

What is Your Worth?

- ▶ Why knowing your worth is crucial to a successful practice

- ▶ How to determine your value per hour

- ▶ Managing time to increase revenue overnight

When you have balance in your life, work becomes an entirely different experience. You develop a passion that moves you to a whole new level of fulfillment and gratitude. This is when you are the best for others and for yourself.

A little secret

I'm going to tell you a secret. A very important secret. A secret most people don't understand. One that I find vitally important. It will change the way you see yourself. It will change the way you practice medicine. All the physicians I have worked with consider this to be an enormous game-changer in their life.

But, first, I need you to write down (on page 24) the five things that are most important in your world.

Don't continue on until you have written down these things. They may take a minute or two for you to think about.

1.

2.

3.

4.

5.

Now let's continue with my secret. If you read the news, scroll Facebook, see the headlines on Yahoo or watch the eventing news then you know the hot word of the moment is *equality.*

Groups around the world are constantly trying to solve this issue. Why are people of different colors, nationalities, and races not given the same opportunities? Why do some people have a better opportunity for education? How do we make it equal for everyone? How can we give everyone the same advantages? How can a person in other countries make the same amount that someone does in the United States?

How can we equalize things?

While these issues are important, we often forget about the one great equalizer in this world.

It doesn't matter if you're a billionaire, a tradesman, a woman, a man, African American or Indian.

Time does not discriminate!

Time can't be purchased, sold or given away. Wealth, age, race, and socioeconomic status have no influence. No one is allowed more hours in the day. Time is one of the greatest equalizers in life.

Likewise, wearing a white coat does not miraculously give you more hours in a day. The only effect your white coat has on your time is how much your time is worth.

How you choose to spend every hour of the day is what will determine the success of your medical practice and ultimately the success of your life.

Can you answer the following questions:

1. What are you worth per hour?
2. How much does Medicare think you are worth per hour?
3. How much do you make per hour?
4. What are your office expenses per hour?

Let that sink in for a second.

Every hour of every day you are worth $2,000 an hour!

Not only are you worth $2,000 an hour, but **Medicare** thinks you are worth $2,000 an hour.

I know what you're thinking….

"This lady has no idea what she is talking about. I've never made
$2,000 hour, let alone from Medicare!"

I am going to use the simple procedure of a nail avulsion you understand how to calculate your hourly worth.

The calculation below is for example only!

How long does it take you to diagnosis an ingrown nail? 10 seconds?

How long does it take you to do a nerve block injection? Not drawing up the medicine, but physically injecting the medicine. 60 seconds, if you are slow. Physically removing the nail adds another 60 seconds.

Total time: 3 minutes or less.

Someone else can:

- ☑ draw up the medication
- ☑ bandage the toe
- ☑ bring in the supplies
- ☑ do your documentation

It takes less than 3 minutes to complete everything you are legally required to do as a physician. This is a low-skill procedure; if you performed twenty in an hour, you would make $2,000 from Medicare. That doesn't even include the office visit fees that might be applicable or over the counter products provided to the patient.

The following example is the national average reimbursement for nail avulsions multiplied by how many patients you could perform in an hour (20 patients).

Income Per Client x # of Clients: $108.36 x 20 = $2,167.20

I am not suggesting for you to do 20 nail avulsions in an hour! This was only to help you understand your hourly worth as a physician.

To calculate your hourly worth as a physician, pick a common procedure you perform in your office. How many minutes does it take to perform this procedure (if you are only doing what you are legally required to do)? How many can be done in an hour? Now multiply that by Medicare reimbursement. This equals...

...your hourly worth as a physician!

Once a physician understands their worth, their habits and responsibilities typically change.

Is writing your own documentation worth $2,000 an hour or would it be better to pay a scribe $15 an hour? What about personally performing cultures, biopsies, drawing up medication or taking x-rays? Ask yourself: Is it worth my time to perform all the minute duties of the procedure? What am I legally required to do? Can someone else perform the task?

You can even take it a step further. Is it worth my time to take that health insurance I always have to do peer to peer reviews on? Is it worth it to do a $300 surgery if it takes an hour? Maybe it should be referred out? How can I practice smarter and more efficiently?

The "do-it-yourself" attitude should start evolving into "is this task worth my time?" "Is it worth $2,000 an hour?

While this concept isn't too complex, many have difficulty understanding that physicians are not only worth $2,000 an hour in the office, but they are also worth $2,000 an hour out of the office.

Everything that you do in your life should be measured against that amount!

Yes	No	
☐	☐	Is eating dinner with your family worth $2,000 an hour?
☐	☐	Is mowing your grass worth $2,000 an hour?
☐	☐	Is playing on Facebook worth $2,000 an hour?
☐	☐	Is saving $200 on your upcoming vacation worth $2,000 an hour?

Naturally, there are a lot of things you will do that you will not be reimbursed for. No one is going to pay you $2,000 an hour to eat dinner with your family. But if you believe that is vital to the health and success of your family then it is worth $2,000 an hour. If this time brings you peace, happiness, and a sense of balance, it is worth it.

Now, let's examine mowing your lawn. Some people love to mow their grass it gives them peace and a sense of comfort. It is revitalizing and fulfilling. Go ahead and mow your grass. However, is it worth the $2,000 an hour if mowing your lawn is the worst part of your week or causes stress and frustration, is it worth $2,000 an hour? No! It would benefit you to pay someone $60 to mow your yard rather than waste your time doing it. If you wouldn't pay someone $2,000 an hour to do a task, then it is time to find someone else to do that task.

Now is not the time to get stuffy about how much you're worth and refuse to do anything beneath you. However, it is time to develop habits and sort your priorities to fall in line with how much you are worth.

Go back and look at your list of the 5 most important things in your life. What are you spending time on and what are you not? How can you change that?

Growing up, I struggled horrifically with Algebra 2. I remember sitting at my dining room table with both my Mom and I in tears and my Dad incredibly frustrated. My parents were trying their hardest to teach me math that they had not used in 20 years. Thankfully they quickly realized that I needed a tutor. That it was not worth their time or effort to teach me. Likewise, my most vivid memories growing up are spending evenings at the local Dairy Queen eating ice cream with my family. I remember doing homework or watching television at night and my mother would come in and announce that we needed to go on an ice cream run. As a family, we took vacations to Europe and did amazing things, but it is those trips to the Dairy Queen that I remember the best. Those trips were magical.

Does your child need to pass math to graduate? Are you spending hours trying to teach your 16-year-old Algebra that you forgot two decades ago? A math tutor will cost much less than $2,000 an hour and will cause much less frustration and stress. I would prefer to spend an hour eating ice cream at Dairy Queen with my child. Those memories I have made with my parents and then my children and getting frosties with them and are worth every minute and penny they cost.

You should always invest your time where it matters most.

Do you need to spend more time with your spouse or partner? Is it worth $2,000 an hour for you? Is peace in your home worth the time it costs? I personally think a divorce will cost more than $2,000. Invest time in your relationships, it is worth it.

What about playing games on your phone, social media or cleaning your house? Is that worth $2,000 an hour? Probably not. I once put an app on my phone that tracked the amount of time that I spent on it. It mapped out how many times I put in my password to open it, how much time I spent on each app and how much time I spent talking on the phone, google searching, texting, etc. The results were astonishing. I spent an average of 3.5 hours a day on my phone!

- 3.5 hours x 7 days a week = 24.5 hours a week.
- 3.5 hours x365 days in a year = 1,277.5 hours a year!
- 1,277.5 hours x $2,000 an hour = $2,555,000!

My phone had become a part-time job! Granted, a portion of that time was checking my email, texting the doctors I work with, on texting my assistant. I guarantee an hour or two was spent doing very unproductive things like checking my email fifty times, Facebook, and getting sucked into pointless news stories, etc. Things I thought were only taking a minute or two ended up costing me hours of my time. I don't even get to spend 3.5 hours a day directly with my children. Stop wasting your time doing things that are not worth $2,000 an hour.

Write $2,000 on sticky notes and put them on your bathroom mirror, nightstand, home office, and kitchen. Put a $2,000 an hour screensaver on your phone and computers to remind yourself of what you are worth. Ask yourself continuously if what you are doing is worth your time. You can never get your time back. "Time" is irreplaceable. Don't waste it! Plan your life accordingly, both in and out of the office.

Making your Time Worth $2,000 at the Office

While you are not making $2,000 an hour eating dinner with your family, it is essential to maximize your earning potential when you are in your office. How do you make your time more valuable in your practice? How do you make $2,000 an hour?

The answer is protocols.

Simple measures taken by creating, implementing and following protocols can improve productivity, eliminate wasted time and increase revenue.

Your staff can draw up that injection, take that x-ray, do your documentation, bandage that surgical site, and dispense that brace. They can administer tests, biopsies, and ensure that a new piece of medical equipment is being used correctly. Your staff can free up your time to see more patients and to practice better comprehensive care. This is incredibly beneficial to your patients and to your bottom line.

The answer is simple if it does not require a medical license to do it and/or you don't love doing it. STOP doing it!!!

Develop the proper protocols that will allow you to do only what you need and want to do. This will allow you to reach your worth as a physician.

If your office isn't running efficiently and your staff does not know how to assist you properly, it is time to make changes that will help them better assist you.

What are the major time wasters in your day?
Write them down and never do them again.

CHAPTER THREE

My Staff is Never Going to Change

● ●

▶ How to implement change in your practice

▶ How to make the change stick

▶ How to get staff to change

● ●

I f I had a nickel for every time I heard the statement "My staff is never going to change!" I would be a very rich woman. It's very rare that a person wants to change on their own. Employees especially hate change. It causes growing pains and many times it doesn't last long enough for an individual to make it to 'the new normal'.

You must decide whether you want to continue to live with:

- ☑ lower-income
- ☑ lower quality of care
- ☑ poor communication
- ☑ long frustrating days
- ☑ no progress

Or if you want to create a center of excellence, where you achieve:

- ☑ higher income
- ☑ better patient care
- ☑ excellent staff communication
- ☑ excited to come to work
- ☑ a passion for medicine
- ☑ reduced documentation

If you want to see changes within your practice, the driving factor must be YOU! You can't expect your staff to change if you are unwilling to change yourself. The problems of a practice NEVER just lies in the staff. Most problems start with the owner and management staff. If you don't want to change, your staff is not going to change. If you don't want to change, your practice will not change and there is no point in reading this book.

There is no point in making protocols, demanding change and then refusing to follow them yourself. Think about it. Do you have workers that don't show up on time. How many times are you there on time? Is there a direct correlation? What about leaving work unfinished or not following through with a task? **Employees mimic the leadership that they see.**

Change is difficult. Commit to yourself and your staff to make the change last longer than the typical three weeks. Continue to implement the change even after the staff pushes back, And yes, they WILL push back.

Remember, you are making this commitment to yourself. No one will be there cheering you on or holding you accountable; you are the boss, and you are the leader

Act like one. Be one.

Join a mastermind group or tape sticky notes everywhere to reaffirm your position. Give yourself pep talks in the mirror, or join my monthly mentoring program, www.gotprotocols.com if you must. Do whatever it takes to commit to change, develop a plan and stick to it.

Make yourself accountable.

Learning Can Be Intimidating

People (and employees) stick with what they know because it provides consistency and security. When new technology, equipment, environments, or procedures are introduced, that security leaves. New processes bring new anxiety. Be prepared.

Throwing your staff into new protocols without proper training is the most frustrating and destructive things you can do during times of change. As the physician, it is your responsibility to thoroughly train employees on all new procedures and tools. It is also your responsibility to bring your staff together and write new protocols as a team, getting their input and ideas.

Although the implementation of the new products, equipment or ideas might seem second nature to you, your staff does not have the same amount of education and training as you do. Field jargon, medical concepts, and high-tech tools will leave them feeling isolated. After all, your staff didn't complete four years of medical school and residency.

At least one person on your staff will be afraid or intimidated by the change you are implementing. It is important to come from a place of authority, but also support and empathy. Assure staff that change is difficult, but the result will be better for everyone.

Here are a few specific ways to help your staff transition:

☑ There is always a learning curve. Account for it, and plan your training accordingly, providing staff plenty of time to learn.

☑ When you implement the change, have all materials to follow through on hand.

☑ Keep equipment and supplies stocked. Do not implement changes until the required materials are present and ready for use. Trying to implement the plan before the tools are in the practice can be very frustrating for staff and yourself.

☑ Set aside a specific time to listen to staff concerns. If their problem is something that can easily be fixed without hindering the effectiveness of the whole protocol, be willing to make those changes. If not, provide extra training to better support the staff.

Be Adaptive, But Vigilant

Know the difference between a staff that can't and a staff that won't.

If your staff is having problems performing the new tasks assigned to them, it might be time to revisit the drawing board. Communicate about the parts of the protocol that are hindering their ability to complete their work. Assure them that you will pass no judgments for their lack of prior knowledge or experience. Remember: not all parts of the change will work. **Be adaptive!**

Although you need to be compassionate and understanding, remember that you also need to be vigilant for those who are simply unwilling to make changes. To identify this type of behavior, look for constant complaining, dismissal of instruction, or a certain person(s) being at the center of all issues. Sabotaging the implementation or outright refusing to cooperate should be a basis for immediate dismissal.

You must put the practice first.

I refuse to work with people who are not willing to change, and you should too. How could I accept money from doctors who refuse to implement change and improve? It would be a waste of their time, my time and their money.

I expect my clients to hold their staff to the same standard.

Changes in staff, protocols, and work environment are all great endeavors, but none of it will 'stick' without the physician being on board and ready for a change themselves. **Be the leader.**

Reward the staff

Change can be hard and difficult. It can be demanding and exhausting. How do you get everyone on board with implementing the changes? Make a game of it. During a time of growth in my husband's practice, we were trying to reach a new financial level, in order to expand and grow successfully. I needed my staff to reach new benchmarks, implement several new protocols and really push each other to succeed in every stage of development of our practice.

We incentivized the staff with a cruise. In 12 months we needed to reach a certain dollar amount. To reach this goal it would require everyone to follow proper protocols, make sure all money was collected, all billing was done correctly and timely, patient recalls were being done and marketing was done. The nurses and doctors were following treatment protocols and patients where happy. It was not just one person's responsibility, it was the entire staff's responsibility. If someone failed to do their part correctly, no one was going on a cruise. The results? Amazing. No one wanted to let their co-workers down, everyone wanted a paid-for vacation. No one wanted to be the person that made it impossible to reach this goal. The teamwork was amazing.

REFLECTION QUESTIONS

What are the major changes you need to make in your practice TODAY? Where can you start?

CHAPTER FOUR

Always Tell Your Staff Yes!

• •

▶ The best way to support your staff

▶ How to work as a team

▶ How to be a leader in your practice

• •

The Band-Aid must be ripped off for your staff to change. They must understand and believe that the process of building protocols will make their job easier — not harder — and that this change will stick.

How do I get my staff to buy into the process?

If you are not committed, your staff will never buy into it. They know if you are genuinely committed or not. They are anything but stupid.

Begin by asking them what they find to be most challenging at work. More than 90% of the time, it is going to be communication. They don't know what to do, what you want, or what you expect.

Your staff cannot read your mind. It gets frustrating, so prepare to hear some criticism of yourself and do not take it personally. It took me a long time to realize a good leader works with their team — not in front of them.

I had a problem, I hated telling my staff "yes."

I am a Type A personality, above all else, I once believed that everything could be fixed by myself and that depending on others to solve problems was a waste of time. I knew what I was doing, and how to do it best. My way was faster and better. It was my husband's practice, and I was in charge. My opinion was the right opinion, and everyone else's didn't matter.

Because of this belief I held, I lived by two rules: 1) I am right, and 2) if you think you are right, and I am wrong, see rule #1.

My staff voiced their opinions, but I would quickly disagree with them because I knew best. Even when they had good ideas, I would not give them the time of day. After all, if it was a good idea, I would have thought of it!

My staff was awesome. I hired them because they are an incredible group of people that I trust. However, I trusted none of them as much as I trusted myself … because I was always right. After years of living my life by this belief, I finally had a stark realization.

It happened one day while I was sitting at a conference. The speaker instructed us to always tell our staff "yes". I chuckled under my breath. "This speaker has lost her mind," I scoffed. "Always telling my staff yes would be a nightmare." I continued to listen and think, while still laughing internally.

The staff didn't know what was best for the practice. They didn't know the whole picture. They didn't understand that my ability to buy groceries, keep a roof over our heads, and pay my husband's student loans all depended on how well the practice did. They didn't understand the late nights, the worry and the stress of starting and running a business. I had skin in the game they did not. Therefore, I knew what was best for the practice. I always knew what was best for the practice they did not.

I continued to listen to the lecture and decided that I would test her theory, so I could prove her wrong. Plus, I am always willing to take on a challenge. I decided to disprove her approach at our next protocol building session. I was only going to say yes to my staff. I would listen to any ideas or thought they blurted out. I even told them beforehand I was going to agree to everything they asked. This was going to be fun!

It was our best meeting to date, and it completely changed the way I viewed the people I work with.

When I recited this to them at the beginning of our next meeting, they looked at me skeptically and mumbled under their breath that it would never happen. Then one person finally made a suggestion and my staff realized that I was actually going to say yes.

> **Suddenly, my employees became more encouraged and empowered than ever. They began to bring up problems that I, as their supervisor, was unable to recognize from my position.**

Now, I know what you are thinking. "I can't say yes to everything my staff says! They will want something we can't afford, or change our workflow, or cause more problems on my end. They will want to give out free braces or want to paint the waiting room purple. They will want more vacation and more pay!" Instead of simply saying "yes", consider the power of "Yes, but…" When you say "Yes, but…" and you follow with your concern, something incredible happens; the staff thinks through the problem and will either provide a solution or rescind the idea entirely and give another suggestion. At the same time, they feel heard and validated and will continue to give suggestions. Be prepared: their suggestions will be amazing! More heads are always better than one.

Often, my "Yes, but..." inspired staff to solve a problem in a way I never thought of. This allowed us to continue to grow and improve as a practice. It allowed my staff to solve problems on their own. I no longer had to fix everything because this created the autonomy they needed to thrive.

Protocol sessions changed, office meetings changed. Instead of me being in control and dictating what happened, I asked the receptionist her opinion on what happened when patients checked in. I asked the MA what problems she anticipated with the new protocols and how long they anticipated it would take them to do XYZ before the physician entered the room. I was now asking their opinion on what needed to happen in the clinic and taking their advice, even if I did not always agree. I would play devil's advocate and have them think of all sides of the problem and see what solutions they would come up with. If I wanted a different answer, I would help them to understand why it was a better protocol or process. The result was amazing. They felt like they had skin in the game. If the new protocols, ideas, or plans failed, they had failed. They wanted to be right, so they did everything in their power to make the new policies work!

> I learned something from my staff that day: I'm not always right. Sometimes, other people know better than I do. Just don't tell my employees. Or my husband

---

What are some ways you can empower you staff?

What is stopping you from saying "Yes?"

CHAPTER FIVE

Write it Down

- ▶ Why communication is your #1 Priority
- ▶ How building protocols syncs your practice
- ▶ How protocols make patients safer

Mrs. Jones, age 72, arrives for her 11 A.M. appointment on Tuesday. She is coming to get a refill on her cholesterol medication.

The Medical Assistant:

- ☑ escorts her to the exam room where Mrs. Jones shares she has a sore throat and is not felling well
- ☑ takes vitals
- ☑ notices that Mrs. Jones temp is elevated to 101.5 degrees
- ☑ writes a quick note in the EHR
- ☑ documents the vitals
- ☑ leaves in a hurry to do an intake on the next patient

The MA assumes the doctor will look for labs and check on the sore throat she documented in the chart.

As a physician, you are running an hour behind and you are worried about the last patient that you saw that needs to be admitted.

You:

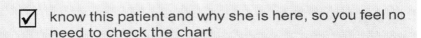 know this patient and why she is here, so you feel no need to check the chart

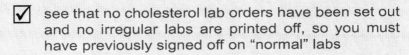 see that no cholesterol lab orders have been set out and no irregular labs are printed off, so you must have previously signed off on "normal" labs

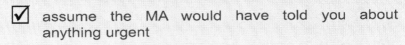 assume the MA would have told you about anything urgent

You briefly ask her about her grandkids, not actually listening to her reply. As she continues to talk about her 2-day-old grand baby, you quickly get on your EMR and authorize a prescription refill on her cholesterol medication that you assume is working well.

Unfortunately, you don't bother to read the chart notes from your MA, telling Mrs. Jones that you will see her next time - neglecting to tell your staff or Mrs. Jones when that date should be scheduled.

You rush to the next room; thankful the visit was quick. While at the same time, hoping the next visit is also quick because you still need to call the hospital to admit your previous patient.

Mrs. Jones then goes to the check-out desk. Where the assistant reviews the notes and sees Mrs. Jones doesn't need a follow-up or a return visit, so she never asks.

Mrs. Jones leaves frustrated - feeling her issues were not addressed. Likewise, she also doesn't know when to come back. Mrs. Jones never returns.

Additionally, no one checked to see if the previously prescribed cholesterol medication was working properly, so Mrs. Jones is sent out of the office with a prescription that may not have been correct.

This patient was a 72-year-old with possible strep throat who was never tested or scheduled for a follow-up.

Although I'd like to tell you this is an anomaly, it is not. This happens to thousands of patients every day in various settings around the world.

The physician did what he was technically supposed to do, which was to address the main complaint. Unfortunately, poor communication with the medical assistant resulted in a potentially sick 72-year-old, possible strep throat exposure to a new infant, loss of revenue, and a patient that will never return.

When you find out about this error, the first person to get the blame will be the medical assistant.

They should have:

- ☑ looked for lab results
- ☑ asked the nurse to perform a throat culture
- ☑ left a sticky not for you

Your front desk should have known to reschedule the patient.

You will reprimand your staff and get frustrated that you provided poor medical care.

What is the end result? An unhappy patient, unhappy staff, and an unhappy physician.

Your Staff Can't Read Your Mind

They have no idea what they are supposed to do if there are no specific guidelines to follow.

Let's tackle this issue by issue.

First, your medical assistant should always be fully equipped to support you. Being organized and supporting the physician is the most important aspect of their job.

They should have:

- ☑ checked for lab results, and in finding that there were none, filled out lab orders
- ☑ asked the nurse to perform a throat culture

Yes, in a technical sense the medical assistant failed at her job. But the real question is, did they know what to check and what to do? Was there a written protocol that they could have referred to? Were there standard written orders for tests or labs when patients meet specific criteria?

Training your medical assistant(s) on how to best support you, and keeping that criteria consistent, is the most important aspect of their training.

Doctors sometimes balk when I tell them their protocols need to be written down. They say that everything is in their head — why waste your time putting it on paper?

Mrs. Jones (and any of your other patients) are the reason why.

If you do not properly train your staff and have written protocols that are easily referenced, the only person who can truly be blamed for incidents like this is you.

While it might seem effective that you have all your protocols memorized, it is unlikely a staff member will. Protocols allow you to set the standard on how daily procedures are supposed to operate. They allow for this all to be documented and easily accessible to the staff.

If protocols are thorough, when someone comes in with a sore throat and temperature, the nurse is automatically authorized to perform a throat culture. If someone calls in to make an appointment for a cholesterol medication refill, then the receptionist is authorized to send over a lab order for the patient to get the required labs completed before the appointment. The medical assistants are required to always pull up the lab results and print them off for the physician to look at.

Everything runs smoothly because all parties know what they are expected to do.

As a physician, you are busy and steps can easily be overlooked.

Protocols help to eliminate scenarios like Mrs. Jones' from your practice. They also eliminate unnecessary risks and wasted time, streamline communication, and improve office efficiency.

You worry about your patients. You worry about a patient who may need an amputation. You worry about a patient who is dying, or who chooses the wrong insurance and can no longer afford the medication they need. You are human and can easily make mistakes because your mind is thinking about your patients, your family, and your business. Just because you own a white coat does not mean you can't make mistakes. Protocols help alleviate this by making sure your staff is always one step ahead of assisting you.

Hang Them With Pride

Protocols should be posted in staff spaces and reinforced in quarterly training. Writing them down alleviates staff from the pressures of decision-making.

When staff are provided with information and resources to perform their jobs effectively, they no longer take your time getting permission to run routine tests. The protocols essentially let the staff act on your behalf.

A fixed, enforced protocol ensures your medical assistant will leave out throat swabs and a cholesterol lab results in the exam room for you, prompting you to perform the necessary tests.

Using a scribe or a note-writing protocol will provide you with diligent notes and improved communication between you, the medical assistant, and the front desk.

> Detailed protocols synchronize the operations in the office and allow physicians and medical assistants to work uninterrupted and unimpeded. When everyone trusts and uses the same protocols, communication is streamlined, conflicts are reduced, and efficiency is strengthened exponentially. This protects your patients—and your business.

REFLECTION QUESTIONS

What are the Top 10 Procedures done in your office?

1.

2.

3.

4.

5.

6.

7.

8.

9.

10.

CHAPTER SIX

There Is Money in Protocols

•••

▶ How a physician can optimize their time

▶ How protocols save physicians money

▶ Staff and the operations of a practice

•••

I f improved time management, better communication with staff, and reduced medical errors are not enough to convince you of your need for protocols, then the automatic increase in revenue should do the trick. Physicians with well-designed protocols will see an increase in revenue in their first month!

But how?

Do you remember how much are you worth per hour? If not go back and re-read chapter 2.

Imagine you're a do-it-yourself physician.

You:

- ☑ prep you own rooms and do all initial intakes
- ☑ room the patient
- ☑ check vitals
- ☑ do any necessary tests
- ☑ explain all treatment options
- ☑ dispense durable medical equipment and show the patient how to use it
- ☑ walk them to the checkout counter and instruct the front desk associate on when you would like to see the patient next
- ☑ finish your notes and prepare to bill the insurance

Following that procedure, you'll be seeing one or two patients per hour. How much is insurance paying for an office visit? $80-$150? Can you afford to only make $300 an hour?

Sure, the patient might need extra tests and OTC products you carry in-practice, but this isn't guaranteed. Sure, you worked that whole hour, but most of what you're doing can be done by a medical assistant. However, most physicians hesitate when it comes to hiring additional staff. They tell me they can't afford it.

If you find yourself constantly doing things that a medical assistant should be doing while your staff is genuinely busy and running at full capacity, hire someone! But, I can't afford it! Stop making excuses and go back and read chapter 2 "What Is Your Worth?"

Make sure you, as a physician, are only doing what you are required to do (injection, check-up, physical, etc.) In most cases, this should only take 5-10 minutes. Your medical assistants and nurses are capable of completing intakes, vitals, x-rays, cultures, dispensing durable medical equipment, completing paperwork, scribe notes, etc. This will free up your patient time dramatically.

The approach of sharing responsibilities with a medical assistant directly improves the patient experience as well. Physicians will be able to see more patients per hour. Likewise, medical assistants can dedicate more one-on-one time to answering questions and making sure the patient feels heard. Ideally, the patient will have someone in the exam room with them 95% of the time. This tells the patient they have not been forgotten and that their time is valuable. The patient will have been properly trained and instructed on how to complete any at-home care by the medical assistant. The patient knows why they need a certain test performed. They understand exactly when and why they need to return to the clinic. The patient feels valued, heard, invested in, and well taken care of. They will trust and build a relationship with the practice. This breeds practice loyalty, which will breed patient referrals. This can be achieved even if the physician is only spending 5 minutes in the room!

You must be sure that each person you hire is doing exactly what you need them to do at exactly the right moment. The only way to do that is through protocols. Fully followed protocols directly increase revenue in medical practices.

> **By building and implementing a plan to use your time efficiently and effectively in the practice, you can delegate responsibilities to your staff, giving you more potential revenue per hour.**

Scenario

A patient comes in for diabetic management. You notice a wound on the bottom of their foot. You yell down the hall for your medical assistant to bring you the supplies that are needed to debride the wound. The MA doesn't bring in what you want so you yell down the hall again and wait. You are now running behind and are getting upset. You know you should biopsy the wound but you do not have time, you will do it next time. You quickly debride the wound, finish bandaging and refill their diabetic medication. You run out of the room circling off a 99214 and enter the next room.

You Have Forgotten To:

1. bill the debridement

2. biopsy the wound

3. dispense wound care supplies

4. do lab work on the patient.

You lost the Revenue of:

debridement	$124.70
biopsy	$100.91
lab work	$34.86
wound care supplies	$1141.52
TOTALLING	$1401.99

If you had written protocols and policies in place, the room would have been set up with the correct supplies, your staff could have performed the biopsy, dispensed wound care supplies, documented the wound characteristics, taken measurements, drew lab work, filled out all order forms and collected all coinsurances. You would have made an additional $1401.99! Can you afford another MA, yet?

There IS money in protocols.

Much of the patient work will be completed by your office staff.

---

[1]   2019 Medicare national payment amounts for correct CPT.

You, as a physician, must ensure that the work <u>gets completed</u> but that does not mean that <u>you have to complete it</u>. One of the greatest time management skills is knowing when and what to delegate and how to delegate it!

Delegating and outsourcing are not just a matter of getting work off your plate and freeing up your time, they are a matter of trusting someone to get the job done. I am telling you right now that you are probably not delegating enough. Your MA, receptionist or office management can complete the job. Train them, give them the information needed and let them fly!

KEY POINT: There is a big difference between being responsible for getting things done and being the one who must do them. When you realize this, you can save a great deal of time by delegating tasks to other people.

What tasks are you doing that are not worth $2,000 an hour for you to complete?

What tasks are others better suited to perform?

What tasks are you doing that your medical license does not require you to perform?

What tasks do you hate doing?

How are you going to make the change?

When are you going to make the change?

CHAPTER SEVEN

Your Office Is Not a Charity

● ●

- ▶ Why some offices bleed money

- ▶ Keeping records up-to-date

- ▶ How to set billing protocols
    that streamline revenue

● ●

D r. John runs a small Obstetrics practice. He has dedicated patients who come back year after year, but the office has a small staff who deal with lots of last-minute emergency appointments. They are often overwhelmed by paperwork and are constantly behind on billing.

There is an unwritten rule that the receptionists are to check for insurance benefits and deductibles each time a patient has an appointment. Unfortunately, they forget to verify insurance while they're trying to juggle multiple check-ins, scheduling follow-up visits, and making sure each patient walks out with the correct prescriptions. The front office staff believes they are doing a great job because they are collecting office copays on every patient, keeping Dr. John's schedule full and staying on top of immediate paperwork.

Dr. John is incredibly busy but can barely pay his bills. His staff say they don't have time to do their job but he doesn't have the revenue to hire additional staff. Dr. John's office is in a cash flow crunch and he is not sure what is wrong. He figures he just needs to see more patients but he is exhausted after working 80 hours a week. He blames the insurance companies for not reimbursing enough. He is getting burnt out and frustrated. His staff is also burnt out and frustrated

What can be Done?

Fortunately for Dr. John, the data never lies. The problem can clearly be seen in his revenue cycle management. 18% of his patient accounts are 180 days past due. Many owing several thousand dollars from their deliveries and surgeries. 60% of his patient's statements are not being paid within 30 days. 10% of his insurance claims are getting denied because the patient insurance or demographics has changed. The biggest problem of all is Dr. John has no idea any of this is happening.

Collecting copays, billing insurance, billing the patient and hoping the patients will pay is not a good business model. Your practice's cash flow will suffer, and your A/R will spiral out of control. A practice must have written protocols for collecting deductible and coinsurance at the time of the visit.

Consider the following scenarios:

Ms. Barker calls in. She is a new patient with an ingrown toenail. The receptionist asks if they will be processing any insurance on her behalf. She states that she has BCBS. The receptionist asks for her policy and group number when making the appointment. Coverage information is verified, and Ms. Barker has a $4,000 deductible with no copay and a 10% coinsurance once her deductible is met.

Scenario One: See Ms. Barker in the office the next day for a new patient exam and an ingrown toenail removal. The medical assistant will tell Ms. Barker that she has a $4,000 deductible and her office visit and procedure will be due when she checks outs. The physician sees the patient and performs the procedure. Ms. Barker checks out, and the receptionist asks for $226.09 (contractual amount for a 99203 — $128.23, and 11730 — $97.86). Ms. Barker pays and schedules her follow-up appointment. Ms. Baker becomes a life long patient and refers other people to the medical practice.

Scenario Two: See Ms. Barker in the office. No money is collected because the patient does not have a copay. The office bills the insurance but the insurance pays nothing because it all went towards her deductible. The practice then bills the patient and waits for the payment. The practice mails 5 patient statements, makes collection calls, but ultimately never get paid. After a year the billing company writes off Ms. Bakers' balance as bad debt. Ms. Baker never returns to the clinic because she knows she owes money. She goes to the next doctor down the road. Not only have you lost the $226.09, but you've also lost about $50.00 in sending out statements (staff time, printing and postage) and another $30 in staff time for collections calls. You have also essentially paid to see the patient, wasted your valuable time, your employee's time and your supplies. In addition, you've lost a patient and that patient's referrals to your office (an unknown value). Plus you incur an additional cost of replacing that patient.

How do you prevent Option Two?

1. Collect health insurance and policy numbers over the phone for all new patients.

2. Assign specific staff member(s) to check everyone's insurance. Know your patient's deductible, co-insurance, and coverage benefits.

3. Know the various estimated contractual amounts for your office visits and individual procedures.

4. Go over patients in the morning. Staff should know if a patient owes money from a previous visit and what their deductibles and coinsurance are.

5. When a patient is having a procedure done, or durable medical equipment is being dispensed, have a staff member inform the patient that it will go against their deductible and what the estimated cost will be to them today.

6. Collect all money at the time of visit

You can't go to a store and expect to leave with a cart full of groceries without paying. This is no different! Inform your patients of the cost of your procedures and they can make the decision if they want to have the service performed or not.

When patients fail to return to a doctor's office because they owe a balance, many doctors say "good". They don't want a deadbeat patient. But most of the time those patients are not dead beats, they just need to pay their rent, food, and utilities. Medical expenses are the last item on their list to pay. Physicians cannot repossess their car or turn off their utilities. Their medical bills are not a priority to them, but if you collect at the time of service they will pay because they are in pain or need answers.

A Medical Practice is a Business

You want to be a physician and only a physician. You want to see your patients and go home at the end of the day. The last thing you want to do is deal with the business aspect of your practice.

This is not why you went to medical school, and frankly, you don't have the time or a desire to manage a business. Can't your accountant or office managers look at the numbers? Can't they run the business aspect of the practice? Unfortunately, the cold hard truth is that you cannot run a successful practice without knowing your numbers!

Your practice *is* a business. It is your business! This makes you an owner first and a physician second. Whether you agree with this or not, your business is dependent on you being a business owner.

> **If you don't want to be an owner, go work for someone who is!**

Know Your Numbers

It doesn't matter if you are the best physician in the world. You are running a business and to run a successful business, you need to understand the following numbers:

- ☑ A/R report for insurance and patients—this will tell you how long it's taking to get your money.

- ☑ How much money was deposited last month?

- ☑ How many days did you see patients last month?

- ☑ How many patients did you see last month?

- ☑ Amount of charges billed last month?

- ☑ What CPT codes were billed and how many times where they billed?

- ☑ CPT report with payment detail from 2 months ago. (This will show any CPT codes that you are having a hard time getting billed. Does a policy need to change?)

- ☑ Per patient value for the previous three months

- ☑ Expense Report

Most of these reports are easily accessible on your EHR. Your accountant, or accounting software, should be able to provide you with an expense report for the month and for the year.

When I show doctors these numbers for the first time, they are usually shocked at what they see:

- ☑ My patients owe me $100,000?!

- ☑ What do you mean I haven't gotten paid for those procedures?!

- ☑ I thought I was dispensing XYZ more than that!

These numbers will dictate how financially successful your practice can become. It doesn't matter if you are the best physician in the world, if the insurance company and your patients are not paying you or your expenses are out of control, your business will suffer.

Don't run a charity. Know and understand your patient's insurance. If you are not sure how to get started, visit my website or contact me. Create practice protocols that include prices and payments on procedures. Your business bank account depends on it.

REFLECTION QUESTIONS

A/R Numbers: 30, 60, 90+ days

How much money is owed to your from your patients?

How much money was deposited last month?

How many days did you see patients last month?

How many patients did you see last month?

Amount of charges billed last month?

What CPT codes did you bill the most last month?

What CPT codes should you have billed more of?

Per patient value for the previous three months?

Look at your expense report where can you cut expenses?

After looking at these numbers are there things that you need to change?

CHAPTER EIGHT

Prepping for Protocols

• •

▶ First steps to take when starting to build protocols

▶ How to audit your own practice

• •

I n any medical practice, the physician's time is the greatest asset. If the physician spends too much time in the exam room with one patient or spends hours doing documentation, time is wasted, and potential revenue is lost. If you are worth $2,000 an hour and spend 15 minutes here, 2 hours there, 10 minutes here - you have lost hundreds of thousands in a year.

> **Protocols should be built to prevent this from happening as much as possible. A well-written protocol will ensure that medical assistants, front desk associates, and physicians are working together in near-perfect cohesion.**

No two protocols are the same. I often get calls from physicians asking if I can "send some copies of my protocols" to their practices.

This is a common misconception about protocols—especially from those who I haven't spoken to, or haven't seen what my protocols entail. Every practice, physician, and staff are different; so are their protocols. There is no one-size-fits-all office solution. There are never the same protocols.

Therefore, copying down the protocols from this book verbatim and trying to implement them into your own practice is a waste of time. They will not work for your practice—these are just generalized examples. However, along with the step-by-step instructions below, they are a solid foundation you can build your own practice protocols on.

☑ **Audit the Charts:** Before I begin the consultation process with the physician(s), I ask for access into their medical charts and their billing. This allows me to get a better grasp of their practice. What do they treat? How they treat it? How do they bill it? This helps me to assess where the practice is excelling and where they are losing money.

- Are there procedure codes that other physicians are using that this office is not?

- Is the documentation strong enough for what was billed?

- Were the correct CPT codes used when billing?

- Are there codes that were not billed that should have been billed?

- Are all local carrier determinations (LCDs) being followed?

- Are the correct ICD-10 codes being used?

- What is getting paid for, and what is not?

- Would the charts pass a Medicare Audit?

There are many other details that I check for as a consultant. If there are any discrepancies in the above questions, these items will need specific attention when building protocols. Generally, there is a lot of lost revenue found in the audit process.

☑ Audit Workflow: Where is the breakdown in the office? Where is there bottlenecking? When are the patients waiting? What are they waiting for? What specific operations in your office are slow? Do you have the information that is needed when you see a patient? Do you have the supplies that are needed for a procedure? Are rooms set up correctly before you enter? Are you constantly asking your medical assistant to bring you things? Do you have all the forms and documentation available? All these items will also need to be addressed when you are building protocols

☑ Physician Meeting: After I have audited charts, billing, and workflow, I meet with the physicians and practice managers and ask them specific questions about their goals, staff, and the top ten things they treat.

We discuss all new potential practice revenue ideas that I have: new procedures, new products, new durable medical equipment, time-saving measures, cash flow optimization, and the current medical protocols they follow.

Now the work begins, and protocols are ready to be developed.

REFLECTION QUESTIONS

What did you find in your audit process?

Chart Audit:

Workflow Audit:

CHAPTER NINE

Protocol Building 101

• •

▶ Why staff communication is a
  fundamental building block

▶ How building protocols
  syncs your practice

• •

Breaking down roles

Your **staff** is your most valuable asset as you begin writing protocols. You can not write protocols without them! After meeting with the physician(s), observing the staff, and speaking to every staff member, I have the entire staff come together for the protocol building session. It is vital for the whole staff to be there. No excuses.

I begin by telling everyone it is essential they contribute to building these protocols. Their input is needed as to what will work and what will not work. I know the basics, but I haven't spent years in this office. They are the only ones who can tell me the long-term problems that plague their office.

I ask them questions such as:

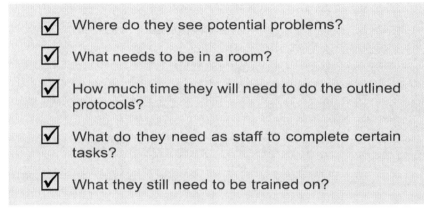

☑ Where do they see potential problems?

☑ What needs to be in a room?

☑ How much time they will need to do the outlined protocols?

☑ What do they need as staff to complete certain tasks?

☑ What they still need to be trained on?

If they are uncomfortable doing any tasks, it is vital they speak up or forever hold their peace. If you are replicating this meeting, make sure to use the technique described in chapter 5.

I start by putting up a large sheet of paper on the wall, so everyone can see what is being written down. Post-It Notes® makes great large sticky paper. I begin with the most common office visit and break it down, thoroughly going through the procedure from the time a patient calls to make an appointment to the moment they check out with the front desk, and received their bill.

The first protocol will take time.

There will be some arguing about who is doing what and how it will be accomplished. *Be patient.* This is usually the first time staff have been able to vent their frustrations about issues in the office.

• •

Physicians are to be at the protocol sessions and be active participants! They can't sit in the corner falling asleep or be distracted finishing documentation. Physicians are responsible for making the final decisions on what tests and procedures will be ordered in every protocol.

• •

These are **your** protocols, and they will change **your** practice.

Make sure they include everything you need. The more specific, the better. A good protocol should include the supplies you need, the tests, the paperwork, and everything else you can think of. Include anything and everything that will make your life easier!

• •

Medical Assistants should support the physician. During the protocol building session, they should be openly communicating with staff and the physician about what they need from them, and vice versa. The MA's responsibilities need to be laid out clearly. They need a guide.

• •

Make sure that you are writing the protocols line by line on the paper on the wall. Everyone needs to see how the flow of the office is organized. This means who does what, how much time is needed and what is needed for each procedure and type of patient. This will be very eye-opening to the staff and to the physician. Rarely does anyone know all the moving parts of an office. Generally, individuals are focused only on their part and specific responsibility.

Making it sync

Always write protocol out in succession.

- 1st visit for broken arm

- 1st follow up visit for a broken arm

- 2nd follow up visit for a cast removal, etc.

This will allow everyone to think in order and decide when things are happening.

Example of a protocol session questions:

- ☑ When a patient calls how do we answer the phone?

- ☑ What information is gathered for an appointment?

- ☑ What are they being seen for?

- ☑ How do we collect insurance information?

- ☑ How and when do we check insurance information?

- ☑ What insurance information are we collecting?

- ☑ Deductibles? Co-insurance? What procedures are covered? What needs prior authorization? Is DME covered? Radiology? Labs?

- ☑ When a patient comes in what do we do at the front desk?

- ☑ What forms are they filling out?

- ☑ What information is being collected?

- ☑ Are co-payments collected now or after the appointment?

- ☑ When an MA brings a patient back what information is she collecting?

- ☑ What vitals are performed?

- ☑ What labs, radiology or tests is she performing before the doctor comes in?

- ☑ What items are needed in the treatment room?

- ☑ What can be discussed with the patient, what can not?

- [x] How do we let the physician know the patient is ready?

- [x] Are test results, labs, x-rays, etc looked at before the physician sees the patient?

- [x] What information is documented in the EHR?

- [x] Is anything pulled up in the EHR or templates started before the doctor enters the room?

- [x] When the doctor enters the room what is being done?

- [x] Is there anything that needs to be assisted with?

- [x] How is documentation being done while the doctor is in the room?

- [x] Once the doctor leaves what is being discussed?

- [x] What questions are being answered?

- [x] Anything being taught?

- [x] What forms need to be signed and completed?

- [x] Any other documentation that needs to be performed?

- [x] What is being documented in the EHR?

- [x] What is the patient paying?

- [x] When is the patient returning for an appointment?

- [x] Why are they returning for an appointment?

- [x] What is the treatment plan?

As you can see there are a lot of different questions that need to be asked and a lot of different answers that will be given. But, it is a necessary step so that all questions, concerns and possible outcomes can be considered. One can not just assume that everyone knows the answers. **Unmet expectations and assumptions can be the root cause of many office problems and hold no place in a medical practice.**

What is needed to make it work?

While you are writing down the protocol and asking the questions you will find that there will be needs. Maybe someone needs to be trained on how to do insurance verifications? Maybe the staff needs to be trained in documentation? Maybe you do not have the supplies that you want for a procedure or a form that needs to be filled out. All of these needs must be written out on another paper. This way they can be addressed. If you fail to address these needs you are setting yourself up for failure.

> **THE ACTION PLAN:** Following a protocol building session, the physician needs to plan implementation, training, continuing education for staff, managing stock, and future protocol building sessions for the treatments that do not happen as frequently.

I never have enough time to help an office create all the protocols they require, but my goal is to build a framework with enough knowledge and experience for the physician(s)to run their own protocol building sessions in the future without my guidance.

To see a protocol session in action,
visit burkmanconsulting.com/protocols

CHAPTER TEN

Protocol Examples

● ●

▶ What a comprehensive protocol looks like

▶ How to build your own protocols

● ●

P rotocols should extend to all interactions between the client and the practice. From the time a patient calls to make an appointment, to when they check out post-appointment, all dealings should follow protocols. Therefore, we must start at the initial phone call when building each protocol.

Having a front desk protocol can ensure that the front desk is getting the NLDOCAT and the insurance information over the phone. Phone Interaction:

 NLDOCAT

● Nature

● Location

● Duration

● Onset

● Course

● Aggravating Factor

● Previous Treatment

Medical Assistant Protocol [20 minutes]:

☑ Insurance Information

☑ Confirm Appointment Time

Front desk associates should ensure that the medical assistant has all the information needed prior to the appointment.

Answering Phone Procedure:
Front Desk Associate

☑ "[Name of Clinic], this is [Name]. How may I help you?"

☑ "Why do you wish to see [Dr. Name]

NLDOCAT

☑ Offer appointment times, date and times (offer only two options at a time).

☑ Input patient name, email, phone number, and address at this time.

☑ "What insurance can I process for you?"

Insurance verification should be done before a patient arrives at the clinic to verify deductibles, coinsurance, and copays. Are any prior authorizations needed? Are there CPT codes that need to be checked for insurance coverage? Does the patient have a balance on their account that needs to be paid? Who is doing this insurance verification? Who is checking balances? When and how is this being done?

Once the patient arrives and is checked in, do you collect copays and past due balances upfront? Do patients need to fill out any special forms prior to being seen? How do you let the medical assistant know that a patient is ready to be taken back? How long does this take?

- ☑ Bring patient back
- ☑ Take vitals
- ☑ Update NLCOCAT
- ☑ Perform procedures needed prior to doctor examination
  - Ex: X-rays, blood work, etc.
- ☑ Bring in heel pain kit
  - OTC
    - Plantar Sleeve
    - Sample of orthotics
- ☑ Braces
- ☑ Consent forms
- ☑ Prepare information for the doctor
  - Ex: Upload x-rays

When a patient is settled in their exam room, what preliminary work needs to be completed? Where is the NLDOCAT being documented? Which vitals are being taken? What needs to be set-up in the room? What labs? Tests? Do x-rays need to be completed before the physician comes in? How much time does a medical assistant need before the physician comes in?

A medical assistant's goal is to make the interaction between the client and the physician as efficient and productive as possible. Pre-approved tests can accelerate the process of treating a patient.

Physicians should aim to be in the room for only the parts they are legally obligated to do. This increases productivity.

Doctor Protocol [10 minutes]:

- ✓ Talk with patient
- ✓ Cortisone injection
- ✓ Prescribe orthotics

Medical Assistant Post Protocol [5 minutes]:

- ✓ Go over the cost of orthotics
- ✓ Give follow-up instruction
- ✓ Sign proof of delivery/consent forms
- ✓ TRC: 2 weeks
- ✓ Walk the patient to the front desk
- ✓ Discuss all completed procedures with front desk/ mention cost

The extent of the role of the medical assistant should be discussed within the office in order to address all concerns and issues such as:

- ✓ Assigning the medical assistant the task of going over treatment plans, answering questions, or reiterating instructions to the patient.
- ✓ Solidifying how much each treatment costs
- ✓ Deciding whether the medical assistant will walk the client back to the front desk, or if there should be paperwork that finds its way to the front desk associate.

☑ Ensuring the medical assistant tells the patient when to return to the clinic (RTC) and give that information to the front desk, as well

The design of the protocols is up to you. Whatever they are, they need to be quickly referenced, thoroughly explained, and posted in every staff room. Pictures of what is needed in a room or for a procedure help tremendously.

Quarterly training sessions (or more!) should be held for physicians and staff to workshop protocols, improving some and reinforcing others. This is the only time a protocol can be changed: when the physician is present.

Staff should keep a record of issues pertaining to protocols or tell the physician directly. They may not take the liberty of changing anything in the exam or waiting rooms without permission. Inconsistency is a sure way to lose current and future patients, as referrals are going to be your most effective marketing campaign.

THE GOALS OF A PROTOCOL

☑ Eliminate Wasted Time

☑ Support Staff and Physicians

☑ Improve Communication and Efficiency

☑ Increase Revenue

Things to Consider When Building Protocols

- ☑ If the condition of a patient falls in line with two or more protocols, which protocol will supersede the other?

- ☑ Who will explain the change to the patient?

- ☑ Be sure to schedule a follow-up to go over the lesser of the main concern.

- ☑ Whenever it is necessary to go against a protocol, the change **must** be documented.

- ☑ If a patient does not agree with the protocol and goes against what the physician has prescribed or ordered, you must record why. This helps protect physicians from malpractice suits.

CHAPTER ELEVEN

Emergency Protocols

• •

▶   Why every office needs an emergency protocol

▶   How to build an emergency protocol

• •

D r. Green ran a very small orthopedic clinic. He was the only doctor in the office, which was run with the help of a Physician Assistant, Medical Assistant, and a handful of the office staff.

The clinic was well-run. There were clear procedural protocols and each employee knew the tasks he or she was in charge of. Almost all appointments to the clinic were post-surgery check-ups, so unexpected events weren't common. Because of this, the emergency protocols hadn't been updated or reviewed since the clinic was opened nearly 15 years before. Nobody in the office gave it a thought since they had never experienced an emergency.

One afternoon a patient, Mr. Smith, came into the clinic for a routine post-surgical follow up. The physician was in surgery, so Mr. Smith was seeing the PA. Mr. Smith suddenly started going into cardiac arrest.

Mr. Smith had blood poisoning, but no one in the room was aware. The PA yelled for the front desk to call 911 as he frantically searched the office for a defibrillator. Unfortunately, it had been moved by the doctor a few weeks before. He hadn't updated the protocol or the staff

Mr. Smith eventually got to the hospital, but the slow response time could have cost his life. An update to the protocol could have saved the clinic an enormous amount of liability.

If you're thinking this wouldn't happen at your office, think again. Medical emergencies happen at every type of practice. In fact, one observational study of rural physician's practices showed an average of eight emergencies per year. Many offices, especially ones with small staffs, are simply not prepared to handle medical emergencies. Here are a few excuses I come across frequently:

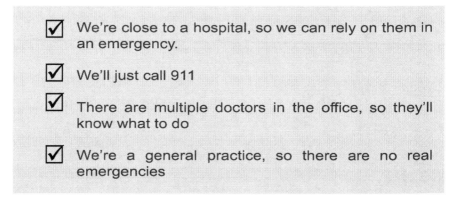

☑ We're close to a hospital, so we can rely on them in an emergency.

☑ We'll just call 911

☑ There are multiple doctors in the office, so they'll know what to do

☑ We're a general practice, so there are no real emergencies

While emergency responders are important links in the survival chain, they do not absolve you of your liability (or responsibility!) to make sure your patients have the best possible outcome in an urgent situation. Every minute counts. Don't put your patients (or your business) on the line.

Hope for the best, prepare for the worst

How do you start preparing emergency protocols?

Think about the basics first. Where are your emergency tools? (Defibrillator, EpiPens, CPR instructions, etc.) Does your staff know the location of this life-saving toolkit? Are they all trained to use these items? If everybody in your office was out at lunch except the person handling the phones, would that person be able to deal with a sudden emergency?

Many physicians think it's a waste to make an investment in emergency staff response training and certifications. All they see is a time and money drain. However, if you knew this training could save even one life, would it be worth it?

Next, think about the specific emergencies that are most likely to occur at your office. According to the American Academy of Family Physicians (AAFP), all offices should be prepared to handle the five most common types of emergencies: seizures, asthma attacks, anaphylaxis, hypoglycemia, and cardiac arrest. Depending on your practice area, you may have more to add to this list.

Make sure you have a specific protocol for each issue that could potentially occur. For example, a protocol for a blood sugar emergency would look something like this:

HYPERGLYCEMIA PROTOCOL[2]

Hyperglycemia occurs when the blood sugar level becomes too high. High Blood Sugar = Blood Sugar (greater than) > 200 mg/dl. High blood sugar can be caused by: not enough insulin, too much food, illness, inactivity or stress. Individuals may display an assortment of symptoms including: frequent urination, increased thirst, increased hunger, lethargy, blurry vision, stomachache, nausea, confusion. Severe diabetic complications develop slowly, over several hours or days. Ketoacidosis = High blood glucose with a disturbance in the body's chemical balance.

---

[2]   www.JDRF.org

- ✓ At the onset of any symptoms, the doctor or highest trained individual should test blood sugar with a meter. Meters are located in the emergency kit A, under the sink of room 12.

- ✓ If symptoms are displayed and a glucose meter is not available. Treat the potential high!

- ✓ If blood sugar is over 240 mg/dl, check for ketones. A ketone test should be performed in the office. Urine is collected in a cup. Then, a strip is dipped into the cup of urine. In approximately 15 seconds, the strip will change color. Use the packaging to read the results.

- ✓ If the individual has HIGH blood sugar have them drink water, 1-2 cups per hour. (no regular soda or juice)

- ✓ If the individual has LOW blood sugar have them drink regular soda or juice (1 cup per hour, more as needed)

- ✓ It is life-threatening if a patient is unconscious. Call 911!

Do not copy this protocol word-for-word. Your protocols must be specific to your office. Each member of your staff should be familiar with your specific emergency protocols and should be informed any time an update happens.

Prepping your emergency kit

Every medical office should have an emergency medical kit on hand. Your protocols should contain a guide to this kit, including where items are located within each kit. Remember, every second counts in an urgent situation.

For general practices, a Basic Life Support (BLS) kit will likely fulfill your needs, although you may opt for Advanced Cardiac Life Support (ACLS) kit, especially if you're far from a hospital or major medical facility.

Because kits contain dated medication they must be regularly reviewed as part of your general protocol. Emergency Management training for staff (ideally BLS and/or ACLS) is also an important step to consider.

CHAPTER TWELVE

Common Protocol Questions

▶ Most common protocol questions

ere is a set of the most frequently asked questions I receive about protocols.

Do protocols change?

Yes, protocols should and will change. They need to be reviewed regularly. In the beginning, they will be reviewed every few months. Otherwise, they need to be reviewed annually.

Many things can affect a protocol. Billing changes occur, a new technology comes, office flow changes, new doctors are hired. It's important to be adaptive and flexible.

Absolutely yes. There is nothing more confusing to staff and patients when doctors do not follow the same protocol. If one doctor always does knee injections the first visit for osteoarthritis, while the second doctor in the office dispenses a brace, patients will have different expectations. It can get confusing to the staff and to the patient. In order to streamline protocols, they must be agreed upon by all physicians in a practice. In addition, the risk of a malpractice lawsuit goes down when all physicians agree to follow a standard of care in their office.

When do I need to hire another medical assistant?

When you find yourself bogged down by routine paperwork and problems, it's time to think about hiring again. Ask yourself these questions:

- ☑ Would an additional medical assistant bring in revenue by dispensing medical equipment, doing more biopsies or running more tests?

- ☑ Are you waiting for your current medical assistant because they are all assisting other patients?

- ☑ Are you doing things that a medical assistant or nurse should be doing?

- ☑ Is there bottlenecking in the office that would be eliminated by having a medical assistant?

- ☑ Are you wasting time?

- ☑ Do you find yourself having to reschedule patients to do things you should have done that visit?

- ☑ Are all staff members busy?

- ☑ If someone calls out or goes on vacation, does the whole office start to crumble?

If the answer is yes to any of these questions, it is time to hire an additional member. Remember how much you are worth as a physician.

Can a medical assistant or nurse perform tests or x-rays before a patient is seen?

Yes. Because the physician is present and prescribes tests, labs, or x-rays to be performed as part of the standard protocol. Various tests can all be performed before a doctor comes in as long as the doctor is present at the office.

I've created protocols, so why isn't my staff following them?

You have spent time developing protocols, but they are not being followed. Why? These are the biggest reasons I see:

● ●

They are not hanging on the wall. You developed the protocols together as a clinic, but guess what? No one is going to remember them. Laminate your protocols, make sure you have added clinical pictures, and *hang them up!* Make sure your staff sees them. Put them in the supply room where they gather their supplies or hang them by their workstation. Make sure they are where your team can reference them.

Protocols are never reviewed. You must review them. You must test your staff on them. You must train your staff on them. Even doctors can forget what was on each protocol. Review them often.

Protocols were never written down in the first place. They must be written down. There is no excuse for this! For those of you that have heard me speak, had me work in your office, or have known me longer than two minutes, you understand this is a requirement. You must write them down. The staff cannot read your mind.

Protocols are never enforced. Just because protocols are developed does not mean they will magically be followed. No one willingly jumps up and down at the chance to change their daily operations. Change is hard and needs to be reinforced by constant reminders and praise.

Supplies are not in plain sight. Many offices stock what they need in a room, but it is never completely set out for the doctor. The whole reason for a tray set-up is to be a constant reminder to the medical assistant and the physician of what must be done. It saves an enormous amount of time versus searching for a product or supply that is supposed to be in the room but is not.

Doctors don't follow the protocols. This is a huge reason protocol fails. Many doctors say it is their staff, but the real culprit usually lies with the physician. They do not change and they do not follow their own protocols. *The doctors must lead if they want their staff to follow.* Don't waste your time developing protocols if you are not going to implement them. If you want to run a successful practice. Follow my three unbreakable rules:

- ☑ Write them down
- ☑ Make them accessible
- ☑ Review and follow them

• •

CHAPTER THIRTEEN

Setting Goals

• •

▶ What a good goal looks like for physicians

▶ Why goals are needed for all physicians

▶ S.M.A.R.T. goals for yourself and the practice

• •

Now what? You have protocols, you have the supplies, you have the staff. *But how is it all going to get done?* If you give a man a bow and arrow then tell him to shoot, the first thought in his mind will be "where?" Not knowing where to aim, the man will just shoot anywhere and at anything, not really caring. Even if he is an excellent marksman with great form, his shooting will be for nothing. He has nothing to aim for and no direction.

What if you give him a target and then tell him to shoot? He will aim for the bullseye. Even if he fails the first time, he will put all his concentration and effort into hitting that target, practicing over and over until he finally hits the mark. There is a greater sense of accomplishment that comes with actually hitting a mark, even after multiple tries than what comes with shooting at nothing.

That is what a goal does: it changes everything. It gives you direction and a purpose.

My goals hang on my office walls. They are a constant reminder of what I must do. My goals are unwavering and unchanging. They are my bullseye, not a dream that changes with the wind. They will be accomplished.

How do I know they will be accomplished? Because I never set myself up for failure. I never set my physician's up for failure either.

All goals (whether for myself or for my clients) have 5 things in common.

They are all S.M.A.R.T. goals.

This means they follow 5 specific guidelines.

• •

Specific: Every detail of the goal should be planned out and decided upon. Building each goal will start with deciding the macro-goal (the result) and then laying out the micro-goals (steps) that need to be taken. The more specific the micro-goals, the easier the macro-goal is to maintain and reach.

Measurable: Benchmarks are a crucial part of goals; knowing when you should be hitting each step and working toward the macro-goal will ensure that you can track your progress. When a goal's progress is measurable, you are more likely to see goals clearly and notice where you need to make improvements before it's too late.

Attainable: You should be the only factor in your own goals; your hard work, actions, decisions, schedule, protocols, and planning should be the foundation for success. Goals that can be affected by other people or outside factors are not attainable by you. You cannot set goals for other people.

Realistic: If you begin by setting unrealistic goals, you will likely fail in achieving them. Unrealistic goals waste time and money. On the other hand, realistic goals consider both time and effort; just because a certain goal is unrealistic to achieve in the next two months does not mean it is unrealistic to achieve in the next two years.

Be honest with yourself about the amount of time and effort it will take to achieve the goal. Don't set up unrealistic expectations. But don't push your deadline out too far. Make it challenging but attainable.

Time Deadline: A goal without a deadline is a dream. There is no way to keep on-task, motivated, and goal-oriented without a hard deadline. Much like the archer without a target, a physician without deadlines for their goals is simply shooting into the sky.

• •

As you should know by now, I love solving problems, I love fixing things, and I love building protocols. But none of this matters unless they are implemented and followed.

I can give physicians the right answers; I can write their protocols I can audit their charts and their notes. The one thing I cannot do is change them. I cannot force them to implement protocols.

So, I do the next best thing: at the end of the consult, I sit down with a physician, one-on-one, and we develop these smart goals together. We decide what WILL be accomplished in 2 weeks, 1 month, 3 months, 1 year, etc. They are all specific, measurable, attainable, relevant, and they all have a deadline.

> **Example: By 2020, ABC medical will generate 2 million in revenue. It is specific, measurable, attainable, relevant, and timely.**

But how in the heck are we going to get there? That is where the micro-goals come into play. How will that 2 million in revenue be generated? Exactly what will cause that increase in revenue? This is what the break down starts to look like[3]:

☑ How many weeks do I work? 48 weeks

☑ Gross revenue goal? $2,000,000

☑ $2 million divided by 48 weeks = a goal of $41, 667 in revenue required each week

How will we get $41, 667 in weekly revenue?

Break down your procedures with how much revenue they generate and how many your office needs to perform each week to create a micro-goal for each.

You may not hit every metric of this goal. You will only be doing and prescribing things that are in the best interest of the patient.

40 new patient visits $120	$4,800
8 carbon or custom AFO's $1,200	$9,600
15 biopsies $100	$1,500
15 custom orthotics $500	$7,500
8 thirty-day supply of Collagen $1,200	$9,600
8 surgeries $600	$4,800
OTC products	$1,500

---

[3] obviously other procedures will be performed.

20 braces avg. $85	$1,700
30 x-rays $45	$1,350
16 ulcer debridement $100	$1,600
20 ingrown toenails $110	$2,200
25 nail care $45	$1,125
60 Established patient visits $65	$4,900

Total: $52,175 x 90% collection rate = $46,954 a week. This is a total of $2,112,930 for the year

You know what you need, now how are you going to get there? You must break down the goal:

The first step in deciding what you want to achieve can be intimidating. Set up five major goals and break them down. These five goals will direct you in achieving what you want. Do not deviate from these goals.

In the next two weeks:

1. I will have the top 10 protocols written and hung in the supply room

2. I will dispense 4 braces

3. I will post an ad for another MA

4. I will have my receptionist check all insurance benefits

5. I will meet with a graphic designer to create advertisements for wound care and AFO's

In one month:

1. My staff will have memorized the office's protocols

2. I will start the office advertising campaign

3. I will take an afternoon to train my staff on how to ast for AFO's so they can take over

4. I will be at 70% of my production goals

5. I will be collecting all co insurance,, deductibles, and co pays at time of service

Continue to make goals for yourself each month. I also recommend having a reward for achieving each goal each month — something to look forward to. This also applies to your staff. When they have something to work towards, they are more apt to be diligent things are done.

Everything that you do should help you achieve these goals. Your ability to accomplish what you want will solely be based on how well you schedule your time. You must learn to say no. If a speaking opportunity, an obligation, or business opportunity is presented to you, measure it against your goals. If it is in line with them and will help fulfill those goals, it is a good opportunity. If it does not truly fit, you must say NO. This will allow you to be open to other opportunities that will be better suited for what you want to achieve. If it is not worth your time don't do it! Delegate what needs to be done.

Physicians love to be busy. However, being busy does not mean you are moving in the right direction. You must only do those things that will help you reach your goals. You have to be able to give your full attention and creative powers to what you love to do and what you want to accomplish.

Changing your practice and working on your goals will be painful and liberating at the same time. Don't stop; make it work. You must commit to this change.

REFLECTION QUESTIONS

Write your goals.
Write what your practice needs to change.
Write what YOU need to change.

CHAPTER FOURTEEN

The Last Word

• •

▶   How to know when protocols need to change

• •

Recently, I was sitting at a bar at the Four Seasons Hotel, watching the bartender hand-squeeze cases of limes, lemons, and grapefruits to use in his signature cocktails. He told me of the cases of limes he hand-squeezed each week for his lime margaritas.

I questioned why he chose to hand-squeeze his juice. He could have used a pre-made mix and saved himself countless hours (not to mention 800 limes).

He stated, very simply, he did it because it tasted better. The quality of the mix was just not the same as the real thing. The customer experience was not the same.

Is it worth the time and effort? To the Four Seasons, it is. To this Bartender it is. He is passionate about watching customers' eyes light up when they taste what he has lovingly created. He loves what he does and his customers adore him for it. Quality and the customer experience is what makes the Four Seasons spectacular. It is what keeps customers coming back and spending money.

What makes your practice spectacular? When someone leaves your office are they amazed by the experience they had? What something sets you apart? When you leave your office at night are you happy with what was accomplished that day? Or do you have a run of the mill medical practice? What red flags is your office waving?

- [x] Every time a patient complains about a long wait or an incorrect bill, it's a red flag.

- [x] Every time you lose a patient who has been coming to your office for a decade, it's a red flag.

- [x] Every time your employees look like they are ready to quit on the spot, it's a red flag.

- [x] Every time you are yelling down the hall for needed supplies, it's a red flag.

- [x] When your bank balance continues to fall, it's a red flag.

- [x] Every time you make a mistake because you're exhausted and overworked, it's a red flag.

- [x] Every time you wake up in the morning and don't want to go to work, it's a red flag.

I've been in your shoes. My husband started a practice from scratch and our ability to eat and pay our mortgage was directly related to whether or not I made things work. I could either go down with a sinking ship, bury my head in the sand or do something about it. I chose to do something about it. Now as a consultant, I have spent thousands of hours in offices exactly like yours. I've watched overwhelmed physicians nearly sink their practices because of routine, but easily fixable mistakes. On the other side of the coin, I've seen practices thrive after fixing their protocols and other things that plague their offices. I've seen physicians spend more time with their families, take home bigger paychecks, and lead happier lives after implementing simple changes.

The choice is yours. You can go down with the sinking ship or you can make things spectacular.

Make the change. Run your practice instead of making it run you. Read and use this book.

Develop and write office protocols. Train your staff to use protocols and collect money at the time of the visit. Know your numbers, how much you are worth, and your long-term goals. This will allow your passion for medicine to return.

> **Being passionate about your job and staff executing protocols, this will give your patients an experience that will make their visit spectacular.**

In return, they'll be as loyal as a Four Seasons guests. There are no excuses. Running a medical practice is difficult, but you can overcome challenges with help from Burkman Consulting. I have proven solutions to help you achieve the results that your practice needs.

PHYSICIAN RETREATS:

Need to recharge and get questions answered? Get ready to relax and take your practice to the next level. Once a year Burkman Consulting hosts an annual retreat. Imagine four glorious days of incredible food, relaxation, and brainstorming. Enjoy luxury accommodations in a 5-star private location, while indulging in the cuisine of world renowned private chefs. Prepare to relax and rejuvenate with massages, golfing, ropes courses, beach walks, private pool/ hot tub, and a fully stocked bar, all while brainstorming with other attendees in a private group of physicians.

Enjoy hands-on workshops and seminars that will make your practice soar. The best ideas are the ones formed after-hours in discussions with other physicians. It is a truly eye-opening experience to gather a group of private practice physicians and let the ideas flow. Questions are asked and problems are solved. We all learn from each other's mistakes and successes. No vendors are ever allowed at this all-inclusive retreat. Sign up now to become part of our world-class think tank.

IN-PERSON PROTOCOL BUILDING SESSIONS:

Once a year doctors join me to learn how to build in office protocols. For one day, we will work side-by-side to develop efficient protocols for your office. I will analyze your data and help develop time-saving, lucrative protocols. Together we will develop goals and help you regain your passion to make your practice spectacular. This is always done a day before the yearly retreat begins.

LIVE STREAM CLASSES & ONLINE COURSES:

I offer online, interactive educational experiences with modular training available. This includes hands-on protocol training and web broadcasts. These classes will equip you with the tools and knowledge to effectively change the way your office runs. I also offer virtual consultation for medical professionals and their respective staffs.

IN-PERSON CONSULTATION:

Burkman Consulting specializes in medical practices. I take the time to understand your unique situation and offer solutions that your practice needs. In most cases, I do all the work that is needed. I come to your office and spend 2-5 days in your practice, working one-on-one to diagnose the issues and provides a solution.

SPEAKING & CONFERENCE KEYNOTES:

Who is a speaker if they don't inspire action? Many times, it is a speaker and topic which draws attendance to your conferences. However, nothing is worse than seeing the same topic discussed over and over again. If a speaker fails to give the audience solutions to their problems (or fails to keep them engaged) the overall event usually fails. My presentations on innovative topics have been known to capture audiences. I educate, inspire, and offer concrete solutions to complex problems that many individuals in your audience are facing. I have spoken on national, state, and regional levels. I enjoy speaking to large groups as well as intimate meetings. I have the education and credentials needed for your staff to receive CEU credits.

Problems I Can Assist With

I have deep experience and education to solve the following problems:

- ☑ Cash flow issues
- ☑ Spending your nights and weekends charting
- ☑ Dissatisfied staff
- ☑ Patient equality
- ☑ Confused staff
- ☑ Complaining patients
- ☑ Lack of staff training
- ☑ Per-patient value dropping
- ☑ Not getting paid for what you are doing

My firm can deal with the following issues:

- ☑ Claim, documentation and billing audits
- ☑ Optimization of workflow and alleviate bottlenecks
- ☑ Setup, revision, or production of protocols
- ☑ CPT analyses
- ☑ Help resolve billing concerns.
- ☑ Increasing revenue
- ☑ Mystery patient (come in as a patient to evaluate the practice).
- ☑ A/R and A/P audit

- ☑ Embezzlement detection and prevention.
- ☑ Staff training
- ☑ Goal planning
- ☑ MIPS completion.
- ☑ Complete Confidentiality. We DO NOT disclose whom we have worked with (unless the physician releases it). We DO NOT work with other physicians of the same specialty with-in a predetermined radius.

Ready, set, change

Change never happens on its own. If you wait for someone else to tell you what to do, you'll remain stagnant and your practice will continue to recycle the same issues. If you're ready to implement true change into your practice, visit our firm at www.burkmanconsulting.com. We can help you find a solution that fits in your budget and meets your most pressing needs.

Made in the USA
Columbia, SC
15 January 2022